My Battle With Cancer
(Multiple Myeloma)

By

Stanley W. Morey, Ph.D.

Forward

It seems to be a quality of most men that, after a certain age, they have a tendency to focus exclusively on the needs of their household and don't socialize extensively. Consequently I first came to know Dr. Stan Morey from a distance, as I saw him struggling in obvious pain to walk the driveways and sidewalks of our community with the assistance of his walker, and in the company of a fearsome little dog that seemed to be little more than a wound up coil (with teeth!) I recall in those days wondering if that "broken down old man" (I would later learn that in his world people such as me were termed "pencil necks") was 100 years old, so feeble did he seem. I could not have guessed that I had a front row seat in one of the most startling metamorphoses I would see in this lifetime.

If the state of other similar communities adjacent to ours serves as any example, our community would consist of a collection of human beings living in close proximity without knowing one whit about one another. Our community, however, has proven to be the exception. During her evening sojourns outside to satisfy her nicotine habit, my own mother started to meet people and develop friendships. This led to her introducing neighbors to one another, which has led to the evolution of our community into one where neighbors, as in times long gone, meet and socialize from time to time. And it is from this process that I came first to know of Dr. Stan, and then to know the man himself.

One evening after one of her nightly excursions my mother dropped an old, yellowed newspaper clipping in front of me that showed two bodybuilders standing on stage. I quickly recognized one of the subjects in that picture being none other than Arnold Schwarzenegger with the other looking only vaguely familiar. Placing her finger over that unknown subject, she told me that this was Dr. Stan in earlier years. It was quite obvious that there was much more to this painfully-debilitated man that I could have imagined! She also informed me that Stan had a PhD in physiology, was a cancer survivor, had a long and storied history, and was someone that I would do well to know better.

The centerpiece of our community is our little tree-lined swimming pool. Over the months Dr. Stan's ability to get around began to noticeably improve, and he and I both began to make use of the pool as part of our regular exercise programs. During those chance meetings we had the opportunity to get to know one another well and share a few stories, and I came to know of this remarkable man's journey through life and his truly inspirational fight with the deadliest of cancers.

It was in 2003 that Dr. Stan discovered he was in a late stage battle with one of the most fearsome cancers, and began to address the biggest challenge of his life - the challenge of survival! For those familiar with the story, the perfect metaphor for Dr. Stan's experience is to be found in the wizard Gandalf's battle with the fearsome monster known as "the Balrog" in the book/movie trilogy "The Lord of the Rings". In that story Gandalf describes a battle of epic proportions that took place even as he descended into the bowels of Hell. It was a battle so intense that, when he finally emerged victorious, Gandalf was no longer his old self; he had transformed into "Gandalf the White", a wizard of less formidable physical presence but with wisdom and magic far greater than his former self. When Stan emerged from his battle with cancer he was more changed that Gandalf. He was four inches shorter due to loss of bone, and his bones were so brittle that simply raising his arms above chest height could result in broken ribs. Pain was his constant companion, and it was all he could do to lie down and contemplate the end of his life (a distinct possibility at that time).

I will allow Dr. Stan himself to serve up the details of his transformation to a man who now moves about the community with no mechanical assistance (other than the occasional bicycle) - a man who finds pleasure in each day - a man who is now known to do the occasional pushup or sit-up beside the pool that has been so crucial to his transformation. Dr. Stan's story is one that needs to be told. The tens and hundreds of thousands of people needs it across this world that are battling cancer this very day.

At the risk of using one movie metaphor too many I will close by citing a movie scene that best epitomizes the essence of Dr. Stan's accomplishment in his battle with cancer. It is the scene at the end of the move "The Right Stuff", when Chuck Yeager, in an attempt to push the envelope with an experimental jet, loses control and ejects as the jet crashes into a fireball on the desert floor far below. As the medic and his buddy drove across the desert towards the burning wreckage the medic spied a faint figure in the distance, obscured by the waves of heat bouncing off the desert floor. The medic asked Chuck's buddy...."Is that a man?"

To which Chuck's buddy replied..."Yeah, you're damned right that's a man!"

Richard "Bringle" Bryant
Tampa, Fl.

Forward

Dr. Stanley Morey…what a guy!

I've known Dr. Stanley Morey since he first began his journey to wellness, and it has indeed, been quite a journey.

When I first met Stan he was out walking his little dog, Sammie. One could see him out with Sammie at all hours day and night and always in his comfy pajamas. My heart broke for him after learning of the battle he was fighting and seeing how very frail he was. That little creature kept Stan from focusing on himself so much and was a very great source of pleasure for him. As they walked the neighbors would stop to pet and play with little Sammie, thereby opening the doors to a great social network.
Stan slowly began to interact with others, thus forming wonderful, lasting friendships. I could see him getting stronger and stronger…it was a miracle!

As time passed and I got to know Stan, we would have many interesting conversations. At times he would have short bouts with depression and I would find myself 'preaching' to him about all his blessings, his natural abilities and the fact that he had such a powerful mind and body. I would try to convince him that he had everything necessary to win this battle. In trying to uplift his spirits, I found that I was really helping myself and always went away with a much-improved attitude. Funny how that works!

Well, all that changed and he did become like The Phoenix as he left the ashes of depression far behind. However, it didn't happen overnight. We would have long conversations about health issues. I have always had a profound interest in nutrition, vitamins, supplements, etc. and to my delight, I had found a very valuable resource and I came to love 'picking his brain'. Now I feel as though I have realized what could possibly be considered a degree in nutrition and wellness as a result of our many conversations and his willingness to share his expertise.

I hope everyone reading this book about my dear friend Dr. Stanley Morey and seeing the pictures that clearly depict his progression will be inspired and come to understand that with a good, positive attitude and a determined spirit that you too, can rise from the ashes like the Phoenix. It absolutely can be done!

Zena Enlow
Tampa, FL.

Forward

Throughout his life, my husband has engaged in a healthy, nutritious life style. He was active in sports during high school, studied physiology in college, and was owner and operator of his own health food store and gym. Not only did he practice health and nutrition, he helped others achieve healthy lifestyles as well. When he was diagnosed with Multiple Myeloma, a cancer of the white blood cells, we were both shocked. Our first reaction was one of fear and desperation. Cancer, the Big C, it seemed like a hopeless diagnoses.

Stan was fortunate enough to get a wonderful oncologist and the Moffitt Cancer Center was just down the road from our home. Stan had a procedure done at Moffitt that involved removing some of his blood, cleaning it, and returning it to his body after he had a strong dose of chemotherapy. The months following that rigorous procedure were challenging. Stan was weak and a mere shell of his former self.

Through his own knowledge of health and nutrition, and the amazing support of a former bodybuilder friend who has an extensive knowledge of herbs, Stan set himself on a road to recovery. Slowly, one small step at a time, Stan began gaining back his strength. He made decisions that moved him slowly toward balance and health again. Diet, exercise, and a positive attitude all worked together to return Stan's quality of life and hope for the future. Today he exercises regularly in the pool, walks his Manchester Terrier, Sammi, eats fresh whole foods, and takes herbal supplements. He is a shining example of the powerful effects of a positive outlook, and an inspiration for others.

Gery Morey
Tampa, Florida

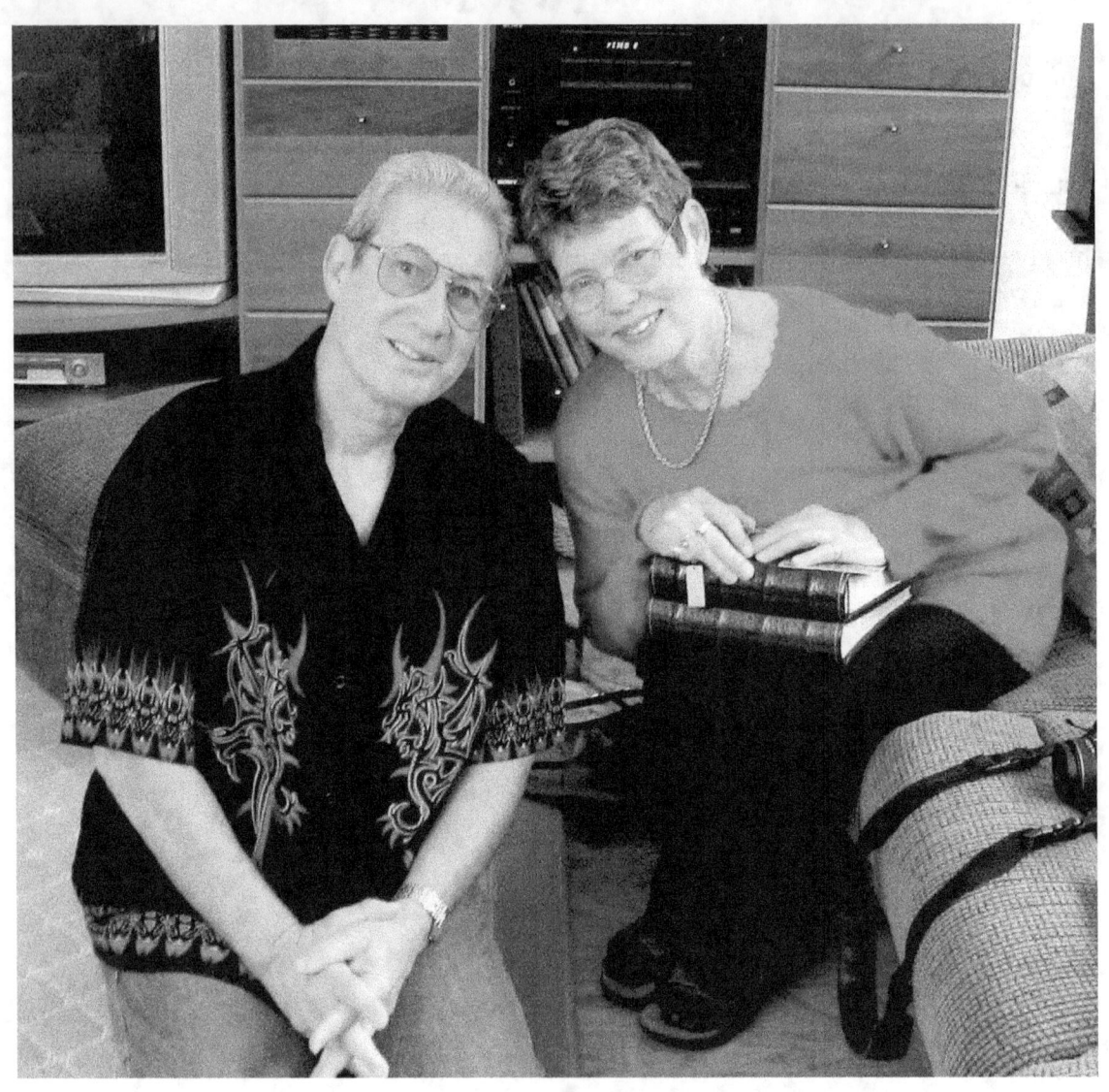

Looking Forward to Many More Years!
Stan & Gery

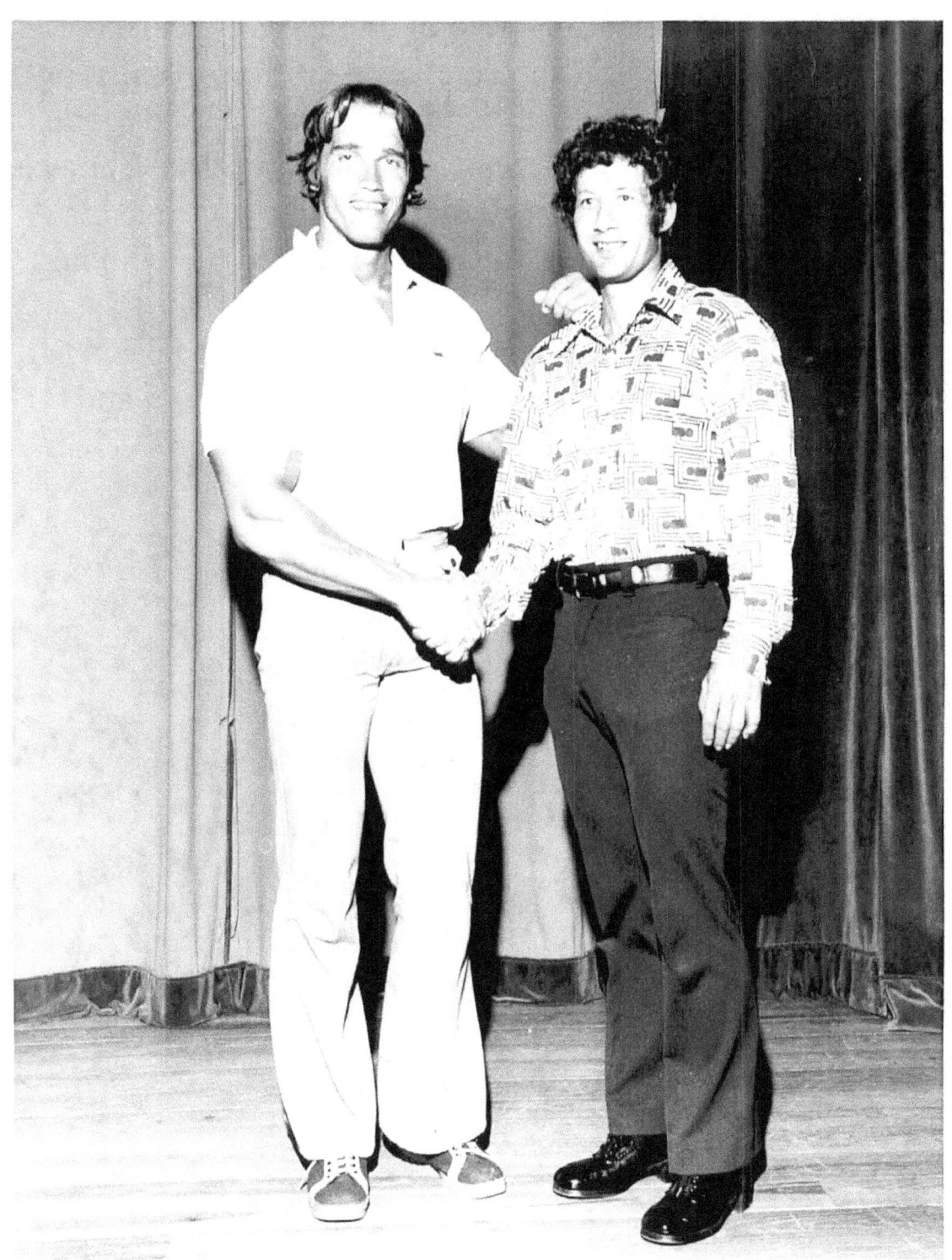

Arnold and the Author in Younger Days

Acknowledgements

I owe a lot of this manuscript to my wife of 45 years, Gery. She stood by during the absolute worst of times. I also owe much to my Manchester Terrier Sammi that caused me to look outside of myself, and care for someone else. She was my constant companion, providing absolute love and friendship. Zena Enlow who always inspired me with her optimism.

I also owe a lot to my friend Robby Robinson (Masters Mr. Olympia) info@robbyrobinson.net for his spiritual and nutritional guidance.

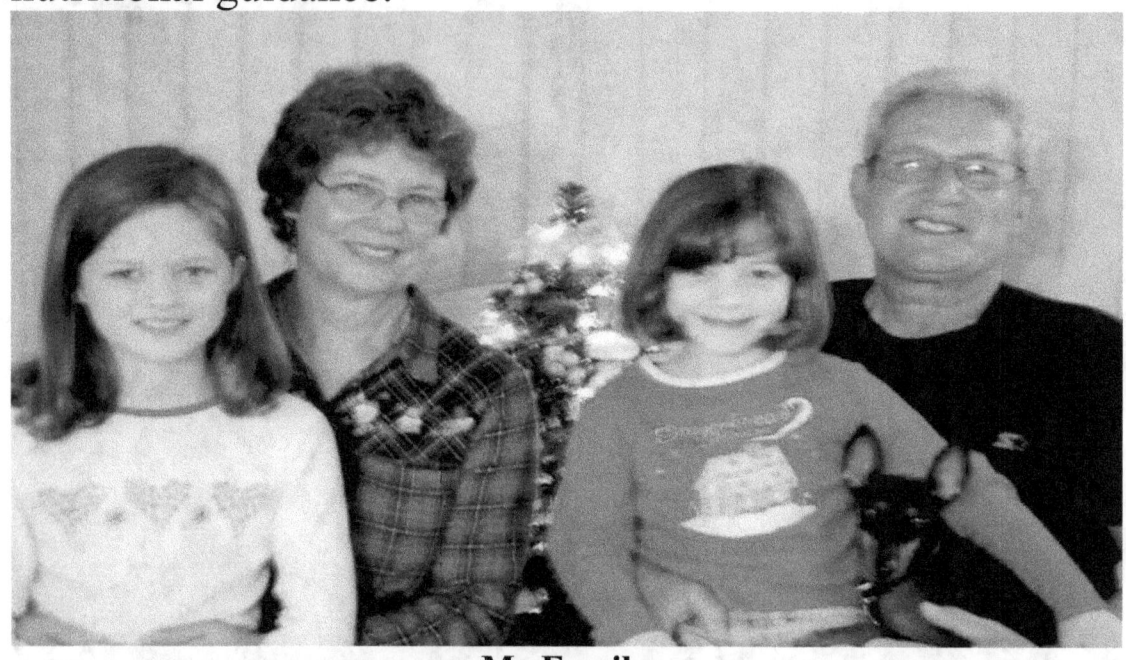

My Family
Left to right : Sarah my Grandaughter, My Wife Gery, Heather my Grandaughter, Sammi, Stanley Morey

I Rose From the Ashes Like a Phoenix

For at least 30 years of my life I was a competitive athlete, playing football, basketball and track. Upon leaving High School I took up Power lifting and Bodybuilding. I became quite proficient in both sports, and was able to win titles in both realms. At this point in my life I felt unconquerable, I was as physically fit as I could possibly be.

When I retired from competitive Bodybuilding, a sport, which I participated in for many years, I seriously took up the sport of bicycling. I purchased a Si 5000 Cannondale Bicycle, which was their top of the line bicycle at the time. I was pretty good, and could average over 22 mph over 10 or more miles. However, I was not Lance Armstrong. I rode a number of Century rides (100 miles), and many over 50 miles. I really was in super condition. My wife Gery also started riding with me, and actually became a bicycling aficionado. It became something we both shared and liked to do. We used to ride every weekend rain or shine we loved it. Our dream was to ride across the United States, a dream I have yet to fulfill.

My first sign of something wrong was when I wanted to give blood, and was refused because I was anemic. I did not think much of it at the time, and felt that it was obviously a mistake. I also started getting slower and slower on the bicycle, my wife was actually starting to ride ahead of me, and during one of my last rides of 30 miles, I barely finished. I was getting tired quite easily. Pain also became a part of my life, but I attributed it to years of bodybuilding and doing heavy squats and dead lifts. It must have been arthritis I thought to myself. I also noted that I appeared to be getting shorter, but again I did nothing. Finally the pain got so great that my wife took me to the emergency ward of University Community Hospital, in Tampa, Florida. They took all kinds of X-Rays, MRI, and CT scans. When the Doctor finally came to tell me the results, he said "Stan you do not have arthritis, however, you have Multiple Myeloma". I was absolutely floored, particularly when my wife asked, "is there a cure". And he emphatically said, **"NO".**

Multiple Myeloma is a cancer of the bone marrow. Usually causing pain in the back and ribs. Pinholes arise throughout the skeletal system. Hematocrit and Hemoglobin levels drop, as does the immune system. I sought the best Oncologist/Hematologist in the area. He started me on a course of Thalidomide© and Cortisone, and Oxycodone and Fentanyl for the pain. But, how was I going to pay the extremely high cost of these medications? Was I going to choose death because of the insurmountable financial obligation? The Thalidomide alone was going to cost me over $4000 per month. I was placed on a **Chronic Disease Relief fund**, which covered these costs. I ended up taking these medications. However, I ended up in the hospital with a side effect from the Thalidomide, which indicated itself as a rash. It took about 3-weeks for this to wear off. Shortly thereafter I started getting really short of breath, and eventually I had to call for an ambulance to take me to emergency again. This time I had a potentially fatal condition called pulmonary thrombosis, or blood clots in the lungs. I was put on blood thinners, and had a Vena Cava filter placed to help with clots. I lay in a hospital bed and was advised not to move. After this episode I became constipated and ended up in the hospital again. At this point my weight had dropped from 198 lbs. to 160 lbs. I had nine compressed and fractured vertebra, 4 fractured ribs, a fractured clavicle, and a lot of pain. I also had developed Osteopenia, which is a lowering of the bone density.

My Doctor gave me a 28% chance of survival, and recommended a new treatment termed Bone Marrow Transplant (BMT), which actually could have ended my life in itself. It was a long time consuming process. I had this procedure done at Moffitt Cancer Center, in Tampa, Florida. This procedure was called an "Autologous Stem Cell Transplant". They used my own stem cells, which were collected after a series of injections to increase their production. After the Stem Cell Implant procedure I could not walk, lost my hair, and was violently nauseas.

 By the time I left the hospital I was a shell of my former self.

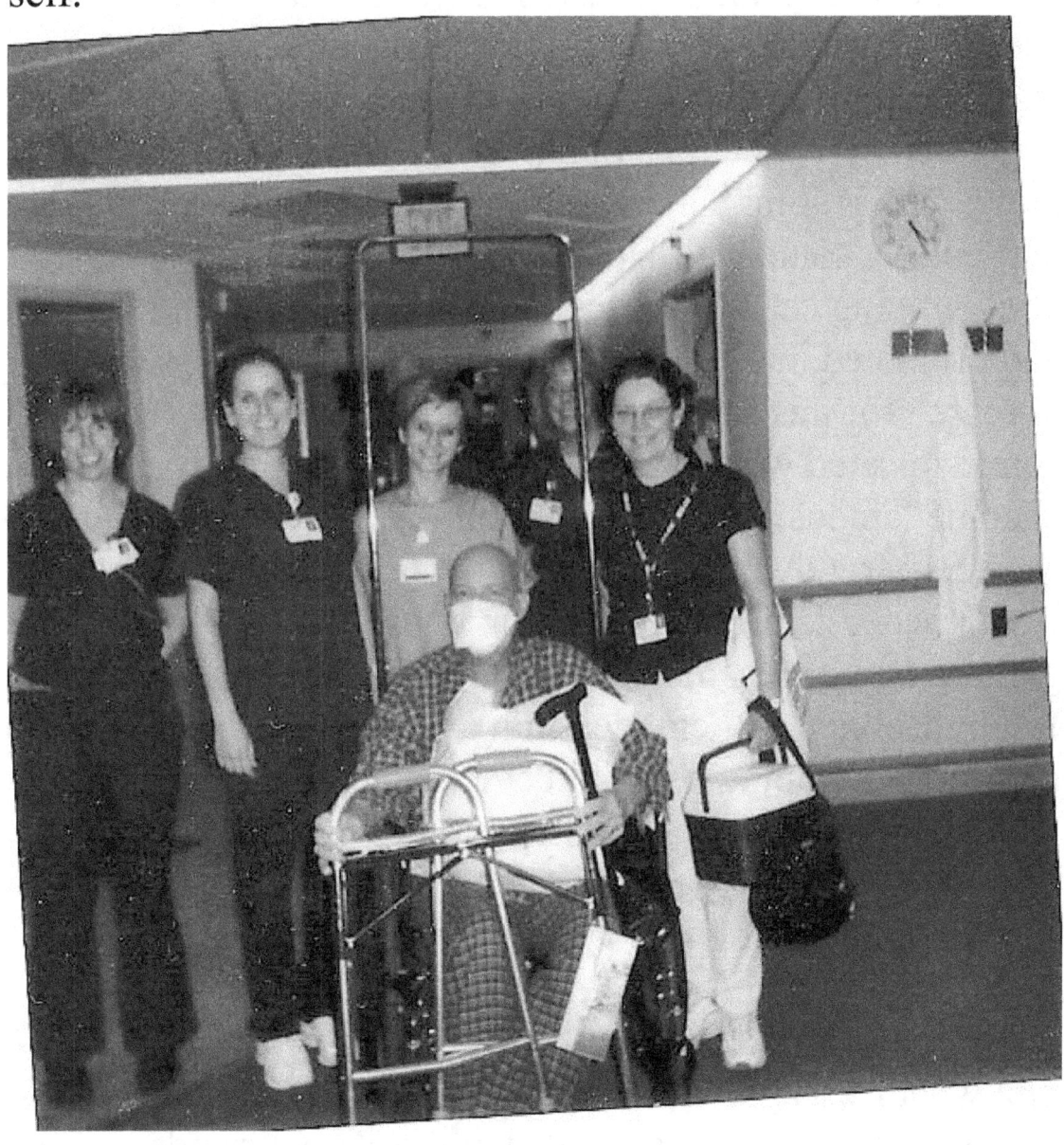

This picture of me was at the time I was released from the hospital. I could barely move, and as you can notice I had lost my hair. I really felt bad.

I actually felt like I was going to die, and in fact at this point I wanted to die. I wondered why I did this? I would sit around not being able to do much of anything, and became very suicidal. I was placed on Paxil© to alleviate these suicidal feelings. These medications in turn caused Erectile Dysfunction, which for me was quite embarrassing, and caused me to become even more depressed. It was at this point that I really made a radical move. I kept thinking and reminiscing about my old days, particularly someone I had helped along with his bodybuilding career. He had won an AAU Mr. Florida I had promoted in 1975. I do not know what possessed me to search for this former friend I had not seen or communicated with in almost 40 years. This individual had become famous in the bodybuilding world, winning the Masters Mr. Olympia; defeating the great Lou Ferrigno who reached fame as the *Hulk* on television. He had garnered the nickname of the "Black Prince". His name is Robby Robinson. I emailed him at an address I found on the Internet, hoping he would even remember my name. And after all the trouble I had with the Weider/National Physique Committee the leaders in our sport of bodybuilding, involving lawsuits and slander, I figured he might want to avoid me. Lo and behold, he did actually remember me, and he quickly answered my email. I told him what I was going through, he told me about his travails, and we quickly bonded and became friends.

However, as we kept communicating he asked me to try the following supplements: An herbal mixture of his design, Glutamine and Bone-Up a calcium replacement (USP formulation by Jarrow Pharmaceuticals). I did not think much of this at first, but I decided to heed his advice. It was also at this time I decided to get a puppy. Sammi was a Manchester Terrier I purchased in the hope of alleviating my boredom, and providing someone else to take care of. She spent all the time with me, and became my buddy. She made me go out and walk her.

At this point I could barely get around. I was taking a drug called Procrit to build up my Hematocrit level, and Zometa infusions to help with my loss of calcium from the skeletal system. My height had gone from 5'10" to 5'6", which was a tremendous compression. I had a procedure called a Kyphoplasty to help aid in the compression caused by the spinal fractures and pain. My immune system was bottomed-out, and my Hematocrit was at an all time low. At this point because of my low immune system, I contracted Shingles, which still bothers me after a few years. However, within one week I found that I could walk about 100 feet with the aid of a walker. After about 4 weeks I started using a 4-wheeled walker. I was able to get around my neighborhood wearing my pajamas. I quickly earned the nickname of the "Pajama Man". Then I got really brave and started walking with a cane. My balance was very poor, and I could not jog or walk unaided. I began exercising in our pool, which helped with my balance, and provided resistance. The exercise program consisted of walking, swimming, and jogging-in-place. I did this every day, even when the air temperature dropped to 39 degrees Fahrenheit. My health quickly improved and I was able to add pushups and sit-ups to my routine. Now I do 20 pushups and 150 sit-ups every day. My neighbors noticed the improvement and could not believe how much I had transformed.

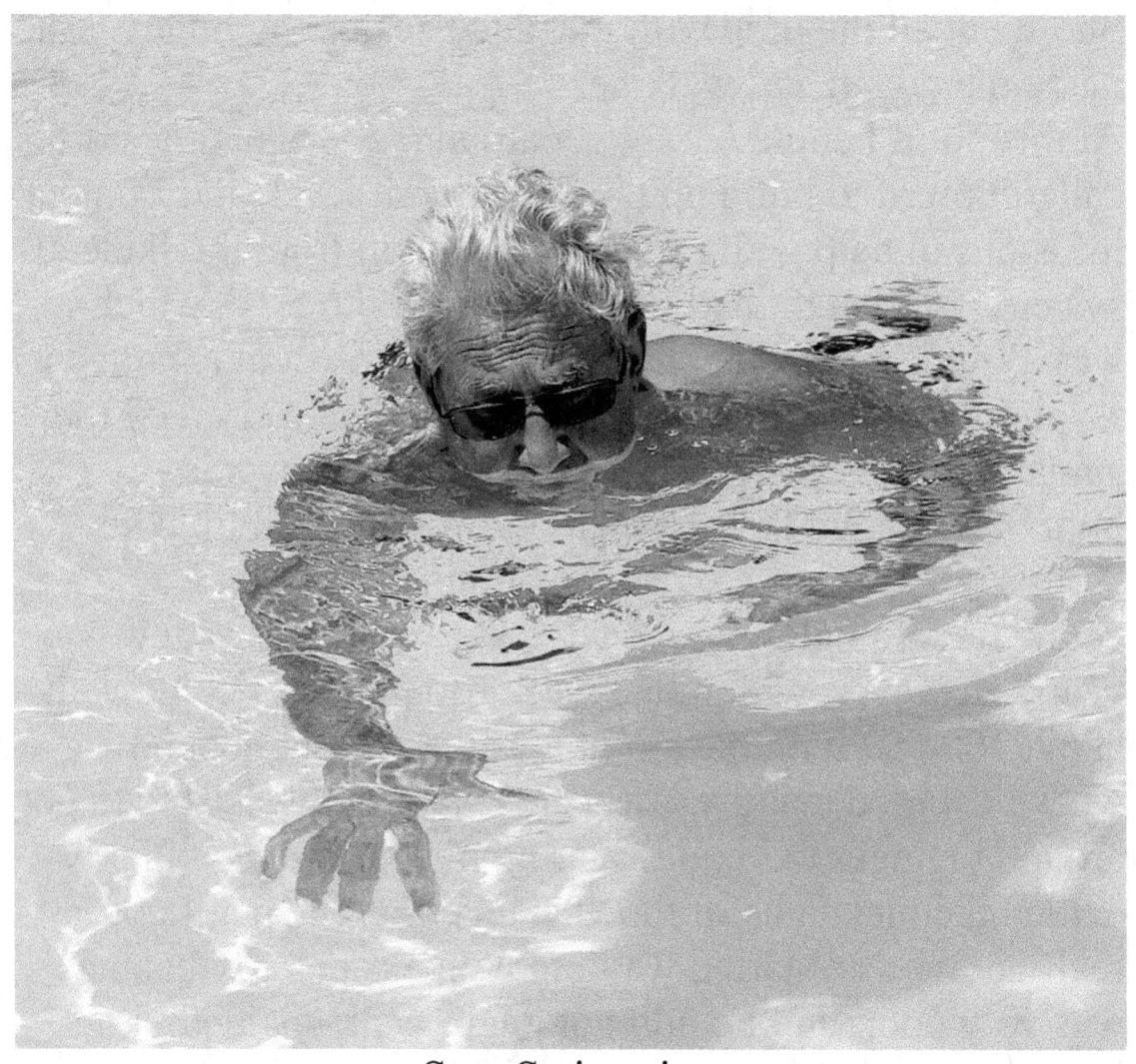

Stan Swimming

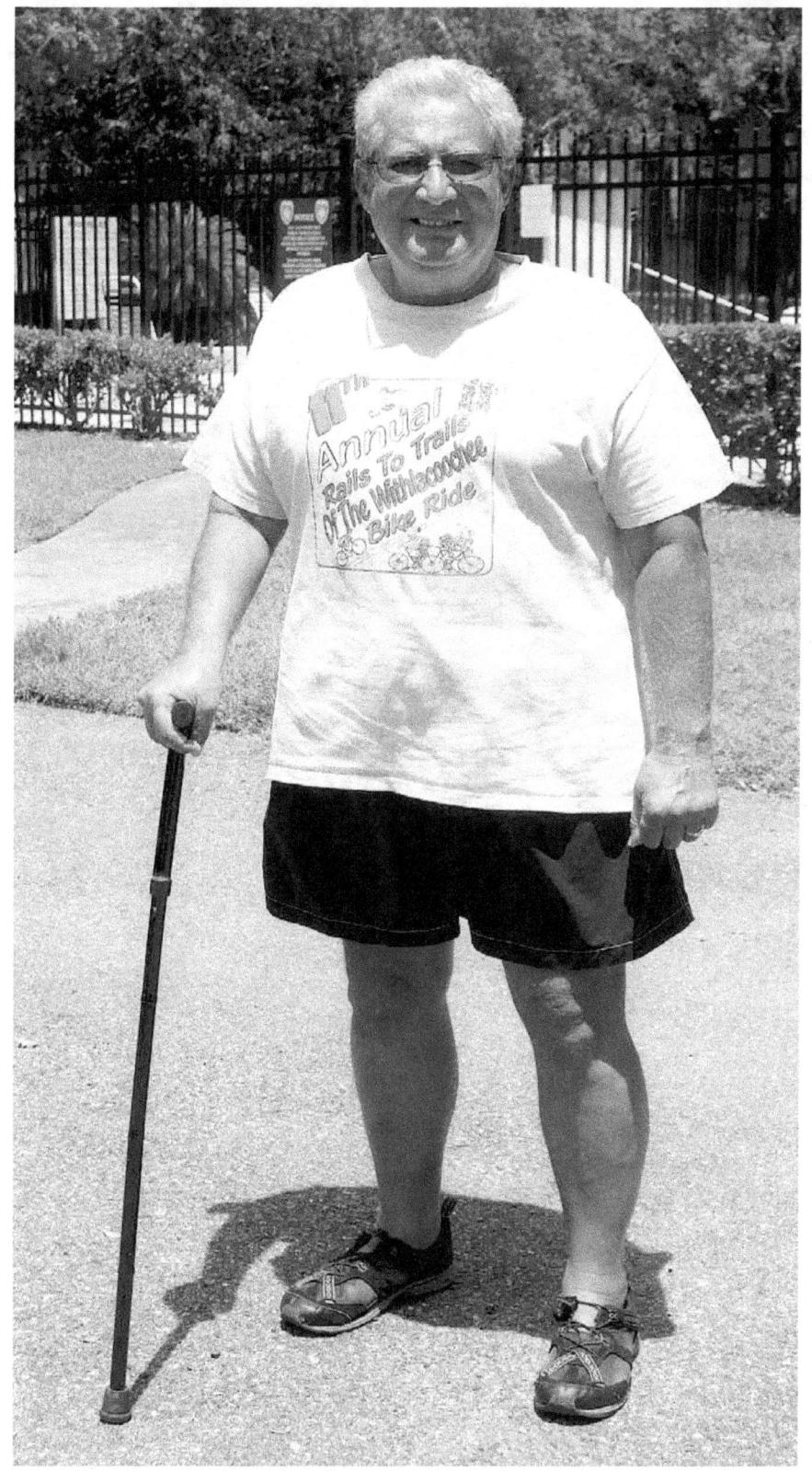

Walking With Cane

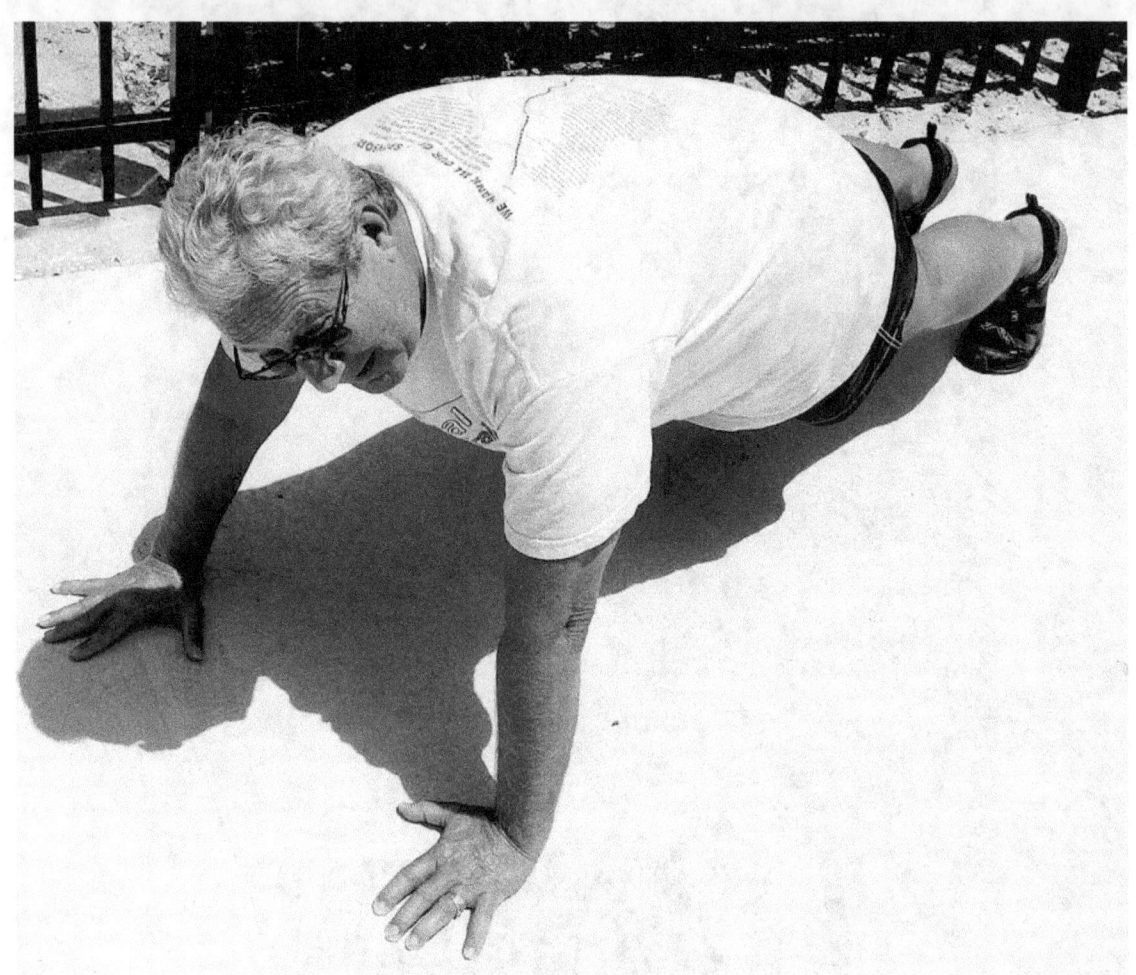

Stan Doing Pushups

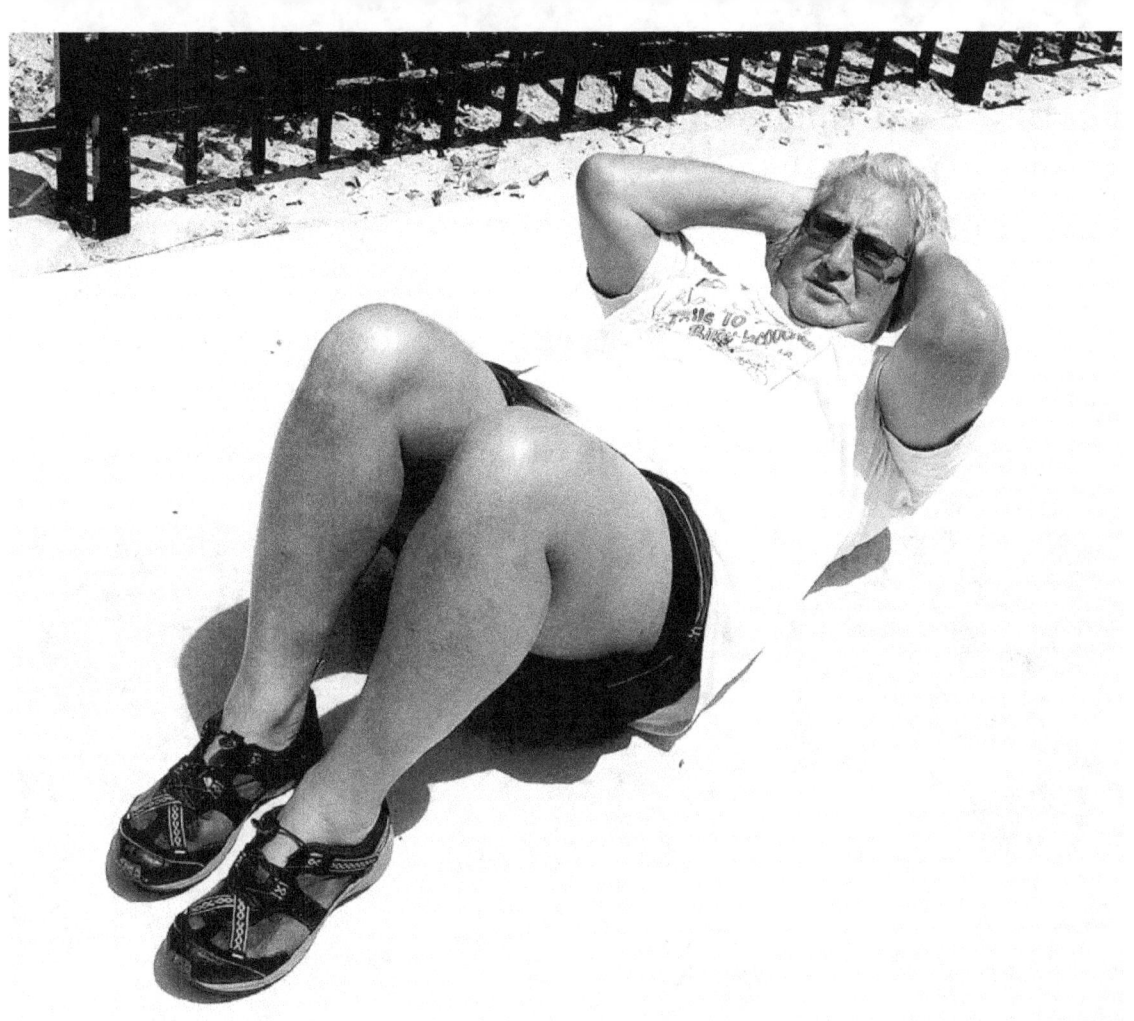

Stan Doing Situps

I am now riding a bicycle, walking approximately 6 miles per day, exercising in the pool, and doing my pushups and sit-ups. I Jog-in-Place for 30 minutes twice daily, which I have found to work very well, and have greatly improved my aerobic capacity. My blood tests indicate normality, my kidney's are functioning well, and my immune system is fine. My Osteopenia is gone; my bone density is now normal. I am living a healthy and happy life in chemical remission.

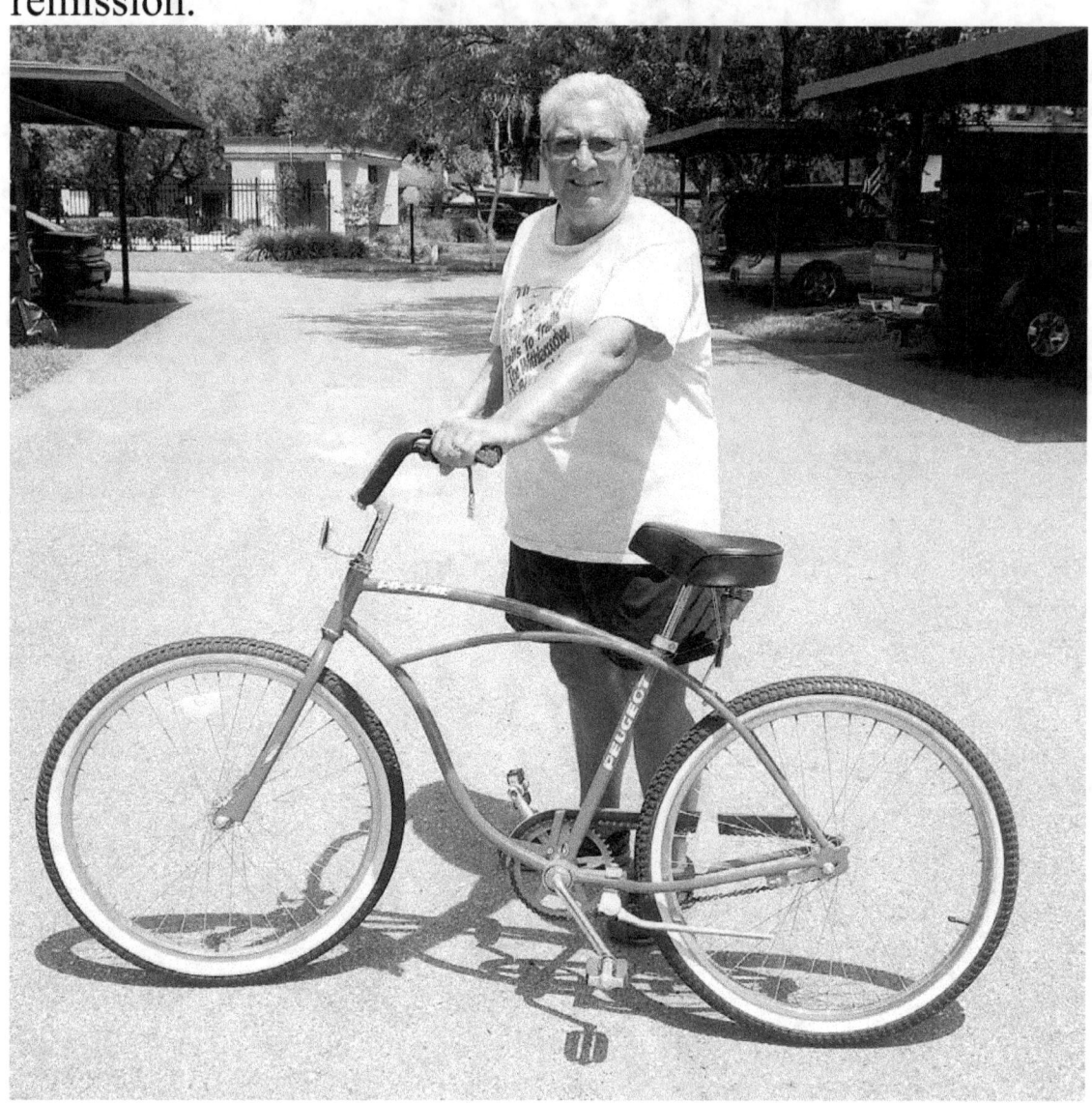

Stan and Bike

As a graduate physiologist I would have thought all of this was due to a placebo effect, however, I also knew that at least 25% of our current pharmacopeia is from herbal materials. What Robby Robinson had suggested really worked, and I have now been able to maintain a healthy lifestyle for over 5 years. I started with an infection rate of 80%. My improvement has been phenomenal. I owe most of that to my friend Robby Robinson and his advice on supplements and herbal formulas. Even though they say Multiple Myeloma is incurable, I am living proof that with spiritual guidance, herbal and vitamin supplementation I am Healing. I recently had a bone biopsy, and was provided with good news that I am still in clinical remission.

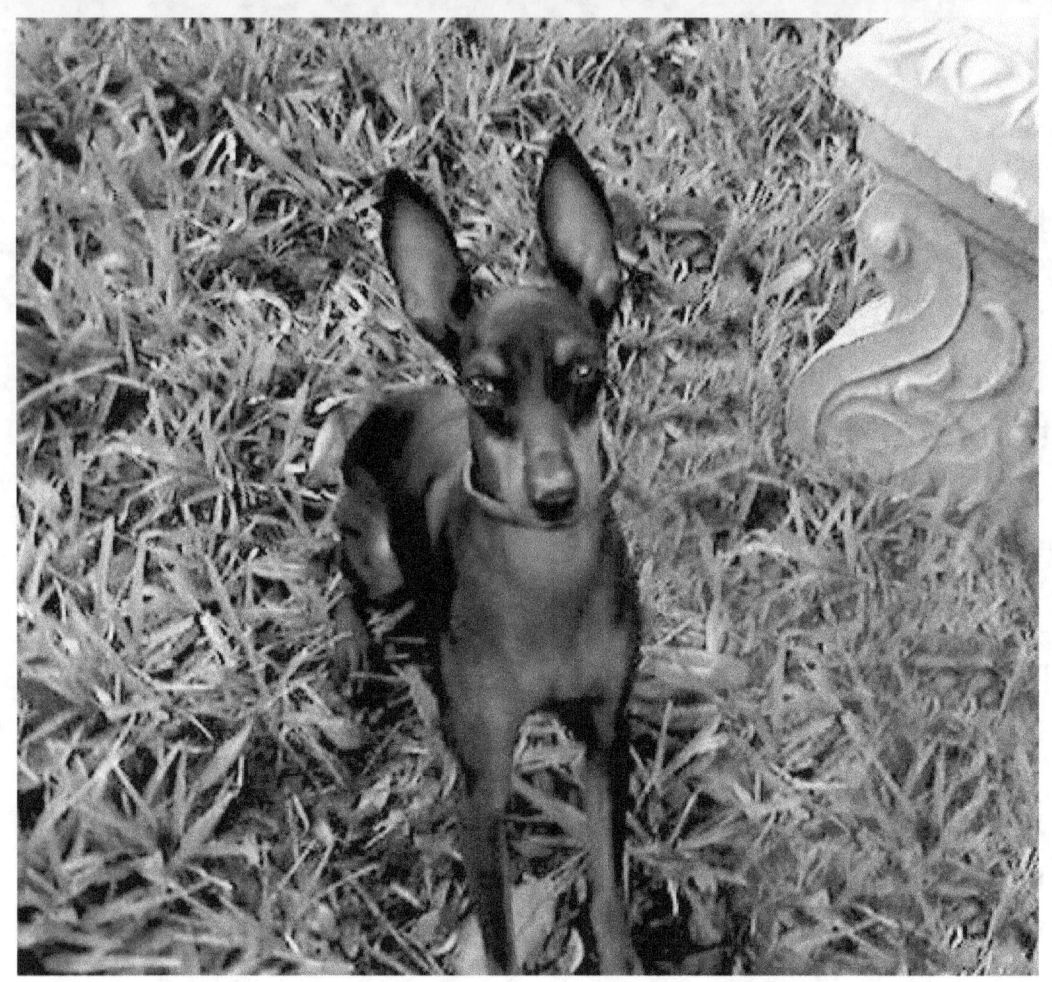

Samantha, one of my saviors.

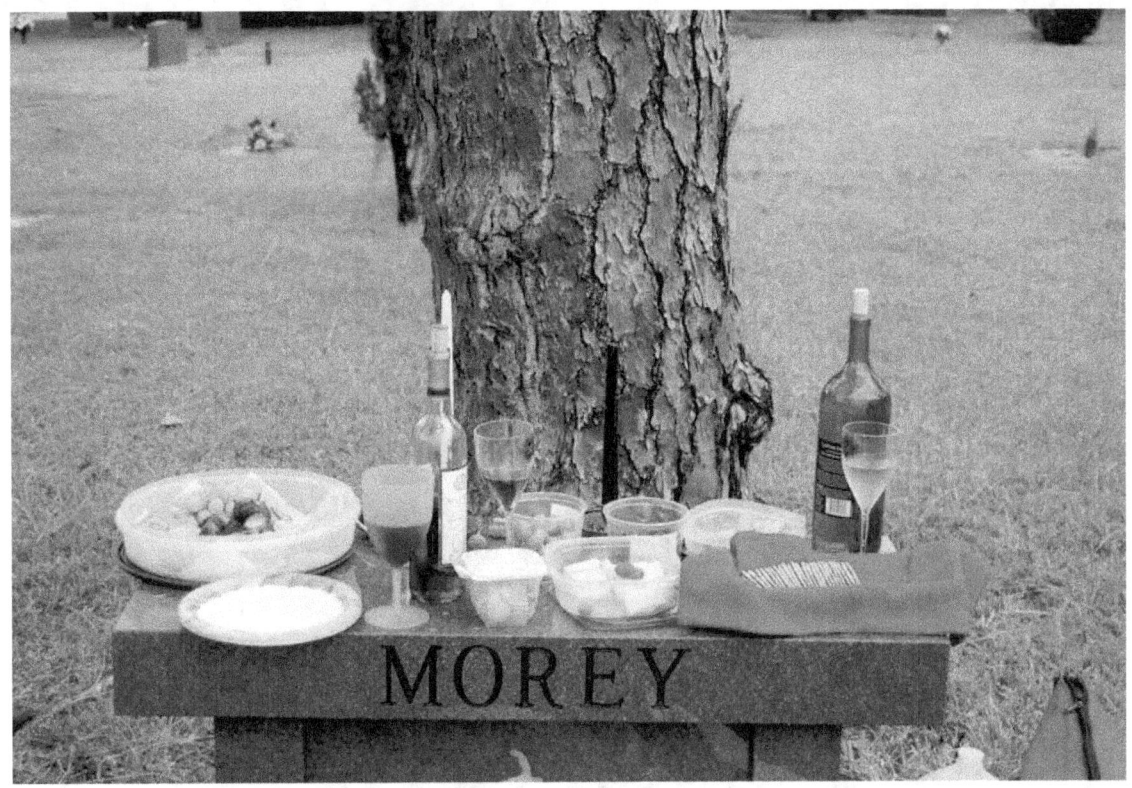

I was so depressed about my life that I purchased a Granite Grave Stone, and actually had a picnic to celebrate my life and passing. I definitely changed my ways after meeting Robby Robinson, and receiving his inspiration. I want to live many more years. I no longer look at this as a memorial to death, but one of life.

Believe and you will succeed!

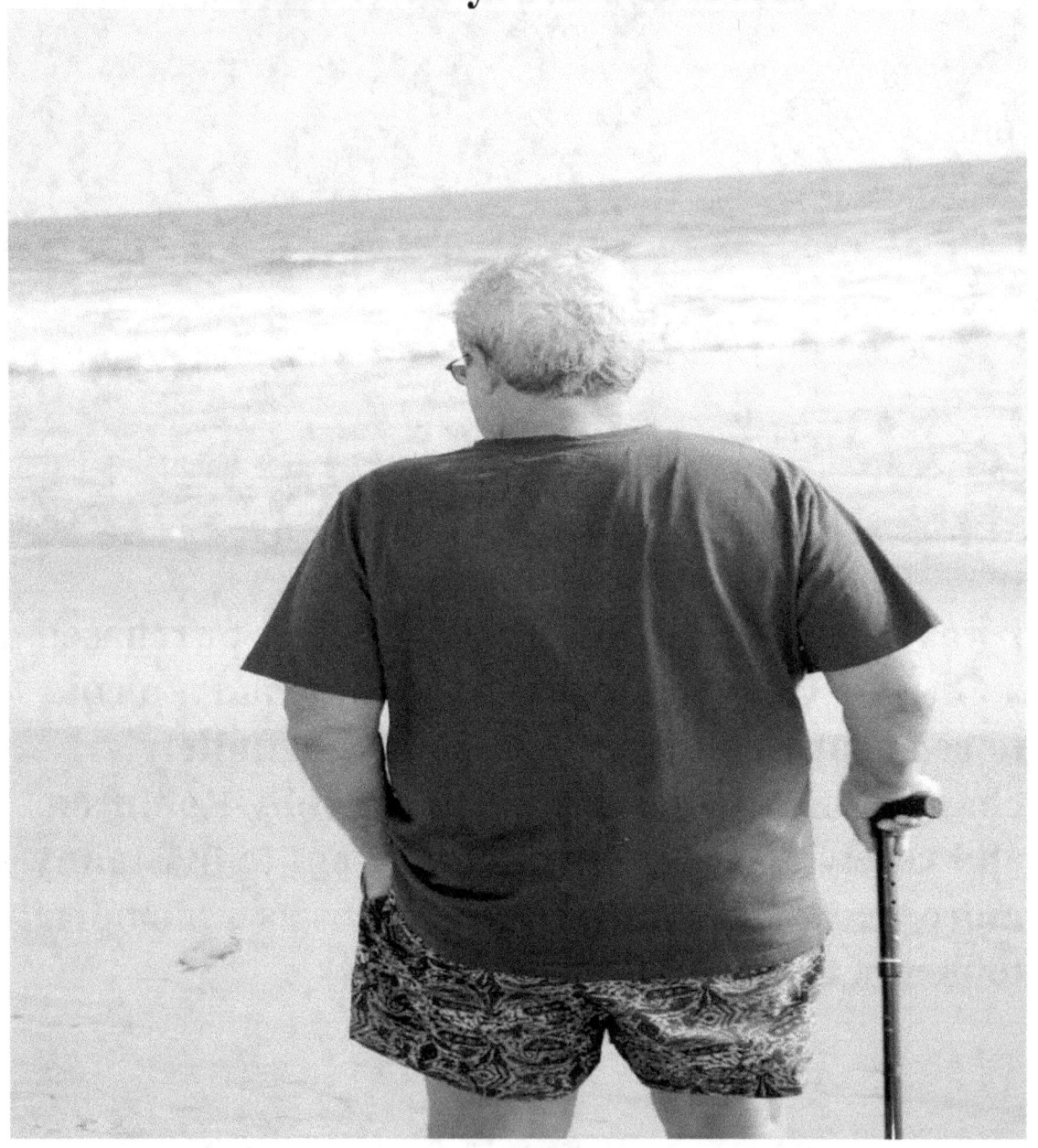

The Author
Stanley Morey

About the Author

Stanley Morey, Ph.D. is an accomplished author, writing many books in the bodybuilding and nutrition areas. He received his B.S. from the University of Tampa, attended J. Hillis Miller Medical School in Gainesville, and the University of South Florida, in Tampa. He received his Ph. D. from the University of the Pacific in 1972 in Physiology. He was also a competitive bodybuilder for many years, winning many local and regional competitions.

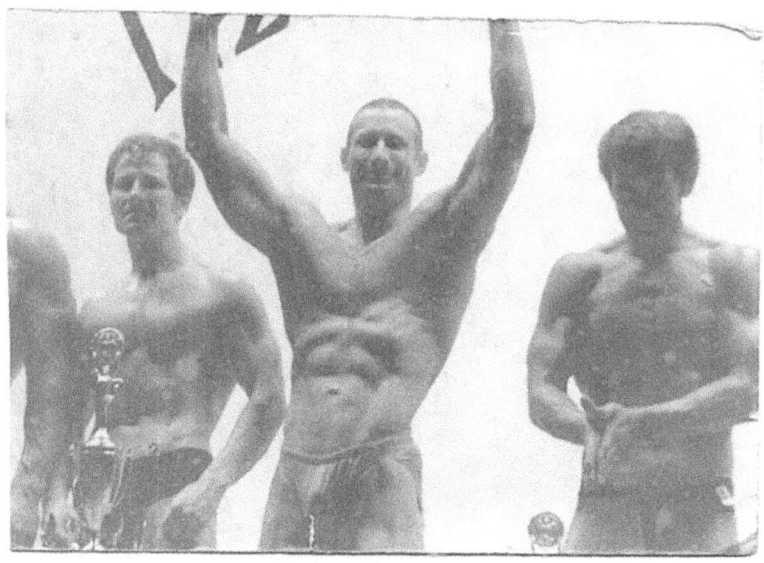

Stan winning Mr. Apollo at age 50